Anti-Aging Skincare Secrets

The Beauty Scientist's Guide to Skincare

Rachel Knight, MSc

DEDICATION

This book is dedicated to my family, and our new addition, Holly. With my brother and his new family in Canada, we can't always be together, but we're always ready to laugh and play when we do. I'm proud we're able to see the world apart, and put the world to rights, together.

How to Use This Book

We'll be taking a holistic approach to youthfulness, attacking signs of age from all angles!

Useful links for each section will help you with further reading, at your convenience. For e-book readers, these can be found at the end of each section, and can be opened by tapping on the link. For print readers, shortened URLs are provided in the Bibliography, split out by section and subject. These start with goo.gl/ followed by 6 digits, so that accessing further information is almost as easy for print readers as it is for e-book readers.

Contents

SECTION 5: HAIR, BROWS, TEETH, LIPS, NECK AND MUSCLE TONE

SECTION 6: AVOIDING AGING

SECTION 7: BUILDING YOUR YOUTHFUL ROUTINE

Introduction

This book gives you the dirt on the multi-billion-dollar anti-aging industry from both a clinical and marketing perspective. Having qualified in clinical research, and gone on to work in healthcare marketing and advertising for several years, I can share with you some tricks on the trade, to ensure that you're not wasting your time or money on fads:

If you are determined to be healthy, happy and youthful- without being ripped off- then update your scam-radar here.

It seems like every week there's a sensational new super food, anti-aging cream, supplement or treatment, and it can be a headache working out which ones (if any) are true. Particularly when scientists are keen to publish small, exploratory studies and advertisers use clever wording, so that genuine products sound the same as products that don't really work. Who has time to work it all out?

It became clear to me how cleverly marketing is put together, during my career as a healthcare advertising executive. Countless rules and regulations exist in healthcare advertising to make sure that medicines claims are backed up with evidence. Even so, *everything* that influences the perception of the audience- words, pictures, statistics- are played with for maximum affect, to make doctors believe that the answer their patients are looking for is in the new drug being released.

Beauty and commercial healthcare clients have infinitely more advertising freedom by comparison to pharmaceutical companies. And the target audience is not doctors, but folk without medical training. So, it's hardly surprising that companies take advantage: *They tell us, their potential customers, what we want to hear to maximize their profits.*

Even though this is understandable in a capitalist society, no one wants to be taken for a ride by marketers claiming to have a new 'wonder' product, food or exercise when they're trying to make a quick buck from a new fad, or the placebo effect.

Using scientifically-backed-techniques, you can build an anti-aging routine that *actually* works, getting more bang for your buck when it comes to anti-aging superfoods, nutrition, creams, exercises, supplements, devices, radiation and more.

My Master's degree in clinical research- a field that specifically looking at how to prove a therapy works- is invaluable in helping me to assess the strength of the claims being made.

There's a specific gold-standard process that is followed to prove that a medicine, device or therapy works, before they can be approved for use by the regulatory bodies, like the FDA in the U.S. or the MHRA in the U.K.

Occasionally, an anti-aging product, superfood, supplement or device might show enough real evidence to warrant being tested in a similar way, so that the medical community can understand it better. In short; we can see what's been proven, and what hasn't.

That's not to say something that hasn't been proven *doesn't work*, but without evidence there's an element of **faith** involved, which you can then decide if you're willing to accept, before you decide whether to invest your time and money in trying it.

Believe it or not, if a skincare product has been scientifically tested, to prove it works better than a placebo (a dummy product to compare it against), the advertising claims will use *very specific words*, that you can easily check for.

Armed with these, and a few key facts about clinical research and the placebo effect, we can feel more confident in future that what we decide to try should hopefully work for us.

Section 1:

How to Understand Evidence

How do you know what to believe when the claims all sound the same?

Marketing Fluff vs. Proof

User ratings and opinion polls

First myth debunked; never take user ratings as a sign that something works. This is where claims such as "87% of women agreed that wrinkles were improved"[1] come in. Why?

1. *The placebo effect* is a strong and proven phenomenon where dummy treatments appear to work because people believe in them. The problem with user ratings is that they usually don't compare a product to a placebo, and if they do, the comparison can easily be biased if the market researcher knows which is which.

2. People are generally nice, and even nicer when given something for free, and giving feedback face-to-face.

---

[1] (*of a sample size of 24 women approached with free gifts while waiting outside the supermarket

Think about it, user ratings are always going to be high, because users have been given free products (they're under the influence of the law of reciprocity), and they don't want to disappoint the lovely researcher who has been so nice to them.

Being honest, how willing would you be to tell someone you didn't like their product when they gave it to you for free, and are staring you in the face? Marketers even have statistics about the percentages of the population that are likely to be genial, and the percentage of people who are going to be difficult. They know who to target first (they call these early adopters) to get the trends going. They even know how age, gender and economic status will affect these proportions.

If you want to be really cynical, they could arrange user testing to be done in the most statistically helpful bunch, like tired young mums, who would love a bit of pampering for the day. Cynical yet?

Cynicism aside, independent of these manipulative techniques, people are generally nice, and are far more likely to say nice things if they know that's what someone is looking for.

3. *Results are cherry picked.* The chances of a user survey having been one question long are teeny weeny. So, out of who-knows-how-many questions, the marketing team have spent hours cherry picking which results to use in their adverts. After that, they retest the message on a new group. How do I know? I've organised and sat in on these advisory boards. Yep, these guys *really* want your money.

Effective ingredients at low concentrations

Many products have very low levels of ingredients such as Retinol or AHA acids that have been proven to improve skin quality, but at much higher concentrations.

The manufacturers are often unable or unwilling to include the expensive active ingredients at concentrations that work, because unfortunately at they often result in side effects. You can only get effective products that have been found to cause medical side effects, from your doctor.

How do you get around this? If you're buying a product, which claims to be effective, make sure that the claims relate to the specific product, *not* to the ingredients. And if the claims relate to the ingredients, make sure that the tests were done on the same concentration that you'll be buying. If not, it might be better to save your money.

Generic moisturisers

The problem that we have with moisturizers, is that basic moisturizers *work*. They raise the hydration levels of our skin, reducing the appearance of wrinkles. Which allows marketers to make their claims.

The question is whether the product making claims works better at reducing genuine signs of age (like wrinkles or marks) than a basic moisturiser, or whether they're using the placebo effect against you. We'll look at this in more detail in section 2.

It's very expensive to run a proper clinical trial on the signs of aging. Market research surveys and user testing reviews are much cheaper, which is one of the reasons they're used much more often. Another reason they're used more often is because most products don't work any better than a generic product, and the manufacturers often know it. They'd much rather put in some nice fragrance, perhaps some colouring, and some chemicals that give the product a nice feel on your skin. But that's not the point. The point is combating the signs of aging over time.

Proven Products

Just when the world seemed so cynical and negative, hooray! There's good news!

If you see the words "proven to work," "clinically proven to work," "proven to be effective" or "clinically effective," you've hit the jackpot! You've found the magic words!

Marketers can't use those phrases, unless the products have been through testing that backs up the claim, which follows a relatively standard process. Ambiguous phrases such as "skin looks like new," "skin is regenerated" or calling something an anti-aging product, is not a straightforward efficacy claim. Without the magic words, I more or less guarantee that a product has not been put through a clinical trial to scientifically assess if it works.

In my experience, not many products would pass up the opportunity to advertise that they've been proven to work, so if you don't see the words, it's likely the results aren't there. If I am wrong, and it has been tested, it probably failed the test, otherwise they'd be telling you about it.

But! Before we celebrate too much, with commercial products- as opposed to medical products- you need to assess what they've been proven to do and how much they work. Scientific testers with biased intentions are still able to design their studies, and make claims in a way that introduces a *lot* of bias in their favour.

Good versus bad trial design

The gold standard trial design for proving if a product works is a 'double-blind randomized controlled trial.' This means that the product under investigation is compared with a control- either a placebo or other form of control- to act as a comparison.

Vitally, neither the subject nor the investigator know who is receiving which product *throughout the process, including assessment of results.* If there are any other people involved in the collection of data, they should also be unaware.

There should be enough people involved in the trial for the conclusions to have been made beyond a reasonable doubt (5% chance of a false positive, 20% chance of a false negative).

Without this type of unbiased evidence, therapies have not been proven in the eyes of the medicinal regulatory bodies around the world, and for very good reason, the results are not trustworthy.

Small significant difference

We're not out of the woods yet. Nearly there, I promise!

Products using the words "clinically proven to work..."? have basically shown that there is a 'significant difference' between how well they work compared to placebo or a comparison product.

But don't be fooled. A 'significant difference' *doesn't* mean a *large* difference. It means a *measurable* difference. Unless the claim tells you how much difference, you have no idea if it's worth your money and time. Would you buy a product for $100 or £100 that had been proven to work "significantly" better than its competitor, but by so little it was barely noticeable?

Tips for summing up product claims
- Don't listen to opinion polls or user satisfaction. They are not reliable for so many reasons
- Look for the claims "clinically proven to work," "proven to work," "proven effective" or varieties of these statements

- If a product claims to work make sure it's the actual product and not an ingredient that's been tested, and if it's the ingredient, make sure you're buying the concentration that was tested

- Look at what signs of aging a product combats, how much it changes them and for how long

Signs of youth

We all want to be in the "looking younger than your age" category (or at least, nobody wants to look older, unless you're underage and trying to get into a bar). So why is it that some women look younger than they really are? And how can the rest of us get in on the secret?

One study by Gunn *et al.* in 2009 set out to determine the features of appearance that determine perceived age, as well as whether or not these features are mainly influenced by our genes, or the environment.

The study looked at two groups, firstly 102 pairs of Danish twins, all female, aged between 59 and 81, and secondly a group of British females between the ages of 45 and 75.

Unsurprisingly, wrinkling of the skin, grey hair and lip height were all significantly associated with the perceived age of the women, independently of each other (meaning that without the other features present, each feature was still significantly associated with increased perceived-age). Facial sun-damage was also significantly associated with how old the women were perceived to be- and was commonly found with skin wrinkles. Recession of hair from the forehead was also a factor in increasing perceived age.

These findings are great news for the readers of this book- because there are several techniques which we discuss later that have been clinically proven to reduce wrinkles, and reduce sun-damage. It also goes to show that "covering greys" and perhaps replacing dulling hair colour with a more vibrant tone is important if we're looking to reduce our perceived age.

The study also found that there was a considerable amount of variation in the perceived ages, which was unaccounted for. When composite images of women who looked young or old for their age were created, the structure of the subcutaneous tissue was found to be partly responsible.

So, are greying hair or wrinkles genetic or linked with your life story? That was also investigated. Greying and receding hair, and lip height are influenced mainly by genetics, and skin-wrinkles, age spots and the appearance of sun-damage are influenced equally by genetics and the environment. Hair thinning on the other hand was found to be more correlated with environmental causes. This is not to say that hair thinning cannot be solely genetic- as genetic pattern baldness can happen in women as it happens in men.

Overall, it was found that the perception of age, is a better biological measure of skin, face and hair aging than chronological age, which is great news as we're about to learn how to improve the quality of our skin.

Other factors that affect the perception of age include the volume and location of fat deposits in our face, with larger volumes of fat sitting in smooth, firm pads around the upper cheeks, eyebrows, chin and covering under-eye troughs. As we age these fat deposits break down, whilst lower areas of the face may accumulate fat, resulting in a drooping appearance.

Body mass index (BMI) has also been found to affect the perception of how old we are. BMI tends to increase as we age, as we carry more weight. The average BMI of an eighteen-year-old female is approximately 20, compared with the BMI of an average 30-year-old female which is around 27. Personally, I prefer a fuller figure, but there's no doubt that a thinner frame is more in line with youth. Before deciding to diet, however, beware! One study performed by a leading cosmetic surgeon found that yo-yo dieting was the leading cause of facial aging in women, higher than stressful life events, such as bereavement, divorce and even illness! Sensible, low-level dieting, toning up and eating healthily can help you avoid facial aging whilst giving you a toned and youthful shape.

Factors of physical attractiveness in women can be roughly split into three camps; signs of youth, signs of fertility, and signs of genetic health. These elements of attraction have derived from and have been strengthened by the fact that they result in increased numbers of healthy, successful offspring. If more offspring survive to have their own families (helped by their genetic health), the selector's genes are propagated further (along with their genes governing mate selection).

This book is about anti-aging, so we're going to cover signs of youth here, but if you're interested in learning about signs of genetic health and fertility in terms of your beauty regime, I have a new book in development for release in 2017. You'll find makeup and styling tips to really help you make the most of what you've been given naturally, and learn how and why you're highlighting or underplaying certain features.

First and foremost, as we've already discovered, clear, smooth skin is key in age perception. We'll continue to learn about how skin quality can be improved in section 2 (skin improvement at home).

Hair colour also begins to change as we age, as the follicles produce less melanin, often beginning in the 30s. Almost everyone loses some hair thickness as they age, both through loss in the number of hairs, and due to thinning of the hair shaft. These changes are not only on the head but can be seen in the eyebrows and eyelashes. We'll consider ways to combat these changes in section 3 (at home hair, teeth and body), along with how you can keep your gnashers looking sparkly and your body giving the right message. So, let's get started....

Section 2:

Skincare Products and Moisturizers

Products you can use at home that are clinically proven to slow or reverse signs of skin aging

Basic Moisturizer

You might have guessed from the previous section, I have bad news about *most* anti-aging skin creams. Most of them do no better job of turning back or halting time than the best of the cheapest moisturisers.

The good news is, cheap or basic moisturisers do prevent wrinkle formation- because wrinkle formation is associated with lower hydration levels within the skin. Moisturisers that work well, often do so because they're better at raising hydration levels in the skin, rather than because any of the active ingredients changing the biological aging processes going on in the skin.

Skin hydration has been found to significantly lower wrinkles and the depth of wrinkle furrows, as found by a 2012 study of 97 women on the influences of skin elasticity and formation of wrinkles by Choi *et al*. A review of skin aging and dry skin by Hashizume in the Journal of Dermatology in 2004 describes how understanding the "basic principles of moisturizer use and application is important for the prevention of skin aging."

If I understand correctly, most people are looking for a product that not only increases hydration levels well (preventing wrinkles forming), but that also works at a more biological level, by increasing collagen production or increasing cellular turn over. *More* than just increasing hydration levels.

If you're happy just to raise your skin hydration levels rather than aim for more, applying frequent, generous amounts of a basic moisturiser that you really like and that seems to suit your skin well, will give you what you're looking for.

Over the Counter Moisturizers that Work

First, I'm going to cover Alpha Hydroxy Acid moisturizers, which have been in use for hundreds of years, but that can cause sun sensitivity, and are less effective than the relatively new Metrixyl moisturizers, which are effective at reducing wrinkles and improving skin quality but have no increased risk of side effects.

Alpha-Hydroxy Acid Moisturizers

Alpha-Hydroxy Acids (AHAs) have been used for centuries to remove dead skin cells, and have also been found to increase the thickness of deeper layers of skin, reduce sun damage and in some dosage regimes, improve acne scarring.

They're naturally found in citrus fruit (citric acid), sour milk (lactic acid), glycolic acid (sugar cane) and others. Remember Cleopatra bathing in sour asses' milk? It had lactic acid in it. It's important to understand the doses needed to get the effect that you want. For treating skin that has been prematurely aged by the sun, products with 8% concentration of lactic, tartaric or glycolic is used and applied twice daily.

For treating acne scars, the acids are used as peels and the concentrations involved increase in strength over time. Unfortunately, some people become extra sensitive to sunlight when using AHA Acids, however, they are more commonly safe than not. Sunscreen and protection should be worn while using them.

When choosing a product, be sure that the concentration of AHAs is high enough to be effective, but beware of high concentrations if you have never used AHAs before.

For example, NeoStrata Face Cream Plus has 15% Glycolic Acid and states that it "is ideal for experienced Alpha Hydroxy Acid users who have demonstrated a tolerance for Glycolic Acid." Peter Thomas Roth Glycolic Acid Moisturizer contains 10% glycolic acid, whilst for beginners Kiss My Face Peaches and Crème AHA Moisturizer contains 4% AHA content.

Alternatively make your own alternative face mask at home to give high enough levels of AHA to work well.

Skin Brightening Lemon and Greek Yoghurt Face Mask and Scrub

½ cup Greek yoghurt (contains lactic acid)
2 lemons (~8% citric acid)
Few drops of white wine vinegar (acetic vinegar)
½ cup cane sugar (for exfoliation rather than glycolic acid- which is virtually non-existent by the time refined sugar has been produced) or regular sugar

Instructions:

1. Squeeze the juice of your lemons into a saucepan and reduce until roughly one third of the volume. Your citric acid concentration will now be about 24%. Don't use this on your face!

2. Allow the juice to cool and mix with the Greek yoghurt, which has a much weaker concentration of lactic acid. Add a few drops of white wine vinegar and stir in the cane sugar.

3. Perform a patch test (as with any topical application that you are trying for the first time) on a small piece of skin on your inner arm and leave for 2 days. If you have no

reaction then you can apply the mixture to your face. Keep the mixture in the fridge while you are waiting.

4. Smooth across your face and leave it for twenty minutes to work.

5. Massage some granulated cane sugar, or if this is too rough some castor sugar, into your skin for a further two minutes as an exfoliator

6. Wash off and enjoy your lovely soft skin!

Alternatively, a milder recipe that also contains AHA, for sensitive skins, is the Blueberry, yoghurt and oatmeal anti-oxidant scrub.

Blueberry, Yoghurt and Oatmeal Anti-Oxidant Scrub

¼ cup blueberries (contains potent anti-oxidants)
½ cup Greek yoghurt (contains lactic acid)
¼ cup oatmeal (contains saponins, a cleansing agent)

Instructions:

1. Mash the blueberries well before mixing together with the yoghurt and the oatmeal

2. Smooth onto a damp face and leave for ten minutes to soften the skin and for the nutrients to be absorbed

3. Wash off using warm water and pat dry

Metrixyl Moisturizers

So, are there any over-the-counter moisturisers without the increased risk of side effects that are better than placebo? Yes. Two products have been proven clinically to work to my knowledge. The first, I am very sad to say, is no longer available, but was called Skin.ny- I wore it religiously after I discovered that it had been "clinically proven to work" and was backed up with astoundingly solid evidence based on a double-blind randomized controlled clinical trial involving multiple solid endpoints. Unfortunately, they've stopped making it and the company have disappeared without a trace, which is very upsetting!

The only other non-prescription product contains Metrixyl 3000 from Sederma, a peptide with proven efficacy in repairing sun-damage in aged skin, and decreasing lines and wrinkles. The serum is sold by the UK Chemist giant "Boots" and is called the "Protect and Perfect" range. Recently the more powerful "Protect and Perfect ADVANCED" serums have been released, which have offered even stronger results. The advanced serums have an increased concentration of Metrixyl 3000, plus a second peptide in high concentrations called "acetyl-di-peptide."

The Evidence

Metrixyl 3000 as an ingredient has been tested by the company that owns the intellectual property rights called Sederma in various studies. Boots have also funded multiple studies directly testing the clinical effects of their serums, which contain Metrixyl.

Evidence collected by Sederma demonstrates that the compound has the ability to repair networks of fibres within the skin, known as the papillary dermis, that are particularly vulnerable to photo aging (sun damage). Papillary fibres are crucial to promote renewed skin and wound healing, which is why papillary dermis repair delivers visible anti-wrinkle benefits. The compound was also shown to reduce further fragmentation of the fibres.

A separate study showed that the compound stimulates various types of collagen proteins. So far, none of this corresponds to *actual* results, such as reduced wrinkling or a more even skin-tone in clinical practice, so at this point it's important to keep digging.

Evidence collected by Boots started off with the collection of small biopsies of skin tissues from 9 volunteers who applied 4 different creams on to a row of 6mm patches on their arms. These 4 were standard moisturiser, weak protect and perfect, strong protect and perfect and tretinoin, a derivative of vitamin A which is prescribed as a topical treatment for wrinkles, sun damage and acne, which I talk about in the next section.

They used tretinoin because they knew that it worked, but only for a few days, as they did not want to risk the usual side effects. Biopsies were collected and compared microscopically to assess the "extracellular matrix", without knowing which was which. Fibrillin microfibrils were found to increase most in the tretinoin patch, and the Protect and Perfect patches scored better than the ordinary moisturiser.

In 2008 Boots increased the strength of the serum to Protect and Perfect Intense and a double-blind placebo controlled trial of 60 men and women aged 45 to 80 years, was conducted. One group received standard moisturizer as placebo whilst the other received the treatment cream and all involved were blinded as to who received what.

After six months of applying the cream 43% of people using Protect and Perfect Intense were found to have clinical improvement in their wrinkles versus 22% of people using standard moisturizer. Dr Richard Weller, senior lecturer in dermatology at the University of Edinburgh, said: "This is, as far as I am aware, the first properly conducted placebo controlled, double blind trial of an over the counter cosmetic product. Boots are to be congratulated for doing this."

Following on from this in 2012 Boots went on to release the Lift and Luminate Day and Night Serum, proven to reduce loss of firmness and uneven skin tone, and in 2014 the Protect and Perfect Advanced Serums were clinically proven to be even more effective at reducing the appearance of lines and wrinkles. After 4 weeks, deep lines and wrinkles were visibly reduced.

Tretinoin and Retinol

The only FDA and MHRA approved topical treatment for wrinkles is a derivative of vitamin A known as tretinoin, and it is available only by prescription. Brand names include Retin A, Atralin and Renova.

It can repair wrinkles, sun damage and acne, and works by increasing the rate of turnover of cells, so that new skin cells are produced and die more rapidly. Common side effects include a burning feeling on the skin, peeling, or patchy light areas appearing.

Retinol is a naturally occurring type of vitamin A, and is often used in many moisturizers available without prescription. These concentrations tend to be very low in commercially available products, because the manufacturers do not want to increase the concentration enough so that the retinol reaches the "therapeutic window" the range of concentrations at which it becomes effective. If they were to do this, the side effects would also begin to increase, and the creams would no longer be able to be sold without a prescription!

You'll notice that very few products state the strength of retinol within them. And so, it's highly unlikely that the products available without a prescription work better than placebo.

Creams to Ignore

As I said earlier, I worked in healthcare marketing as well as doing an MSc in Clinical Research. We advertised pharmaceutical products, and had to follow some very specific rules to make sure we never over-promised.

Commercial advertising, such as for moisturisers follow an entirely different set of rules. Believe me, if there is *real* evidence behind a product, a claim will be made *directly*, and *non-ambiguously*!

If there is no evidence, advertisements will avoid direct statements such as "proven to reduce wrinkles" and will instead make statements such as "skin *appears* younger" "as if restored …" or "I feel years younger" "My skin glows from within…"

Think about this- if the cream did have an additional, measurable effect *on top of* placebo, the manufacturer would have invested in clinical trials in order to prove it, and would have published the results, because the revenue and interest from consumers would have been highly profitable.

And when I say trials, I am not talking about market research tests measuring perception of 93% of 23 women agreed- this cream is better than that cream. I'm talking about double blinded, randomised controlled trials where two groups of subjects receive different products- one placebo and one the test cream- and neither they nor the scientists know which group received which cream.

After a set period of time a scientifically measurable and relevant endpoint will be evaluated and it will be concluded whether a significant (which means measurable, NOT large) difference occurred.

If tested, it is my opinion that almost all creams would be no more effective than placebo. The good news is that the most basic moisturiser, with no special ingredients, does reduce and help to slow the formation of wrinkles. This is what clinical trials testing moisturizers use as a placebo.

If you don't want to spend much money- my advice to you is to stick to a cheap generic moisturiser, one that keeps your face moist, but that suits your purposes in terms of greasiness, keeping your makeup on etc. remember that without any proven anti-aging ingredients, the only anti-aging property is the cream's ability to increase the hydration levels of your skin.

Section 3:

Tools and Devices

Tools for your skin that have been proven to work.
No gimmicks here!

Tools and Devices

There have been incredible developments in at home anti-aging devices that have been genuinely proven to work. From copper-infused pillowcases to infrared, laser and radio devices. It makes me ask what's going to come along next?

Cupron Pillowcase

Ever dreamed about getting younger as you sleep? Interestingly there is a pillow case out there that has been clinically proven to reduce wrinkles. No, it's not witchcraft, it's perfectly scientific!

The fabric of the Cupron pillow is infused with copper. Copper has long been used in bandages and other items because it has both antibacterial properties and it stimulates collagen growth in the skin- hence encouraging wound healing.

In September 2012 Cupron released results of a double-blind controlled clinical trial of 61 people. 30 people used the cupron copper infused pillowcase, and 31 received a pillowcase that was not infused with anything (now you see Pfizer, this is how you give faith to nerds like me that I can trust the numbers I'm seeing- context).

At four and eight weeks after daily use, participants skin was evaluated visually and using imaging equipment that measured wrinkle depth. Roughly a 10% difference between skin wrinkles was measured between the two groups, and this difference continued to rise after the trial.
That's marvellous. So, after two months, wrinkles would be reduced by 10% (on average) and more so after. I will have effectively pressed pause for those two months. But interestingly, the copper never wears out.

You can wash the pillowcase, cut it up, do whatever you like with it- it'll still have the copper inside, pressing pause on your skin (although there are no longer term studies which show whether this result wears off or whether you will eventually catch back up with those where you "would have been" on the aging timeline).

Essentially though, whether facial aging is reversed to a point and then is halted, whether it is reversed to a point and then is slowed, or whether it is reversed to a point and then eventually catches back up, it doesn't matter- you never have to buy it again- it's a one-off investment.

I also bought an eye mask, made of the same material, and gloves for my hands. I'll share a secret- the delicate eye skin by my nose and under my eyes was never coming into contact with any of the material- and so I chopped off the little fingers from the gloves and sewed them to the eye mask in an upside-down "V" so that the material presses lightly against it.
I've had my pillow for about 5 years now, and I love it. I don't know if it works- because I bought it in my twenties at a time when I didn't have any wrinkles to test it on, but it certainly makes me feel like I'm looking after myself.

Anti-Aging Laser Technology

There have been fascinating developments on how parts of the electromagnetic spectrum (that's the spectrum of radiation that ranges from radio waves, through visible light, ultra violet, and up to microwaves and gamma waves) affect the skin.

Different wavelengths are absorbed by different molecules within the skin, which can lead to tightening, damage and subsequent over-repair, or simply improved circulation.

Fraxel

Fraxel lasers are were created to be used in clinics to rejuvenate and tighten the skin. Thousands of microscopic laser rays enter and are absorbed by the skin, causing controlled, evenly spread damage, or burning. This damage to the skin is what prompts the skin to "repair" itself, and in the process of doing so, the skin is improved to beyond the point at which the initial damage was caused- an "over-repair."

These are not the words used by clinics of manufacturers of the devices as "damage" sounds scary! However, when using the device, the effects are similar to very short-term sunburn- except rather than aging you- this type of mild burn is improving your skin!

Following repair- after the skin has "renewed" itself- the collagen density, sun damage and smoothness are increased and fine lines are also decreased.

There are also devices that can be bought and used at home. They are less aggressive, and less effective in terms of benefit per treatment, but the advantage of a lower price and extended period of use, makes these devices an interesting option to consider. Two leading devices are the Philips ReAura and the Tria Age-Defying lasers.

The Philips ReAura is a take-home laser device that is based on the more aggressive clinic-based treatment of Fraxel laser technology. It costs around £800 at the moment, so it's a pricey anti-aging investment! There is a cheaper version called the Tria, which costs £549, which I will go into later.

The hand-held unit uses laser energy to stimulate the skin to renew itself, and by doing so improves several signs of aging. It can be used on the face, neck, chest, hands and arms.

The clinical trial results shown on their websites discuss these results as the end-point of a twelve-week trial with 64 participants, with 81% experiencing a reduction in fine lines, 83% experiencing more even skin tone, and 86% experiencing smoother skin texture. 89% of the group (that's 57 women) experienced one of these 3 improvements. These were NOT opinion polls, but were clinical results. However, the degree of improvement is not stated.

ReAura state that to get the best results, as shown by their clinical trials, it takes 8 weeks for 1 treatment, using the device twice a week. Results are gradual and start to show after 3 to 4 weeks.

The cheaper version of the ReAura is the Tria Age-Defying Laser at £450. Unlike the more expensive ReAura, the Tria has a clearly visible link where the entire clinical trial paper can be downloaded, showing method, explicit results and all.

The trial involved 34 subjects, with each side of subjects' faces being randomly assigned to either daily treatments or biweekly treatments at different treatments levels.

The subjects were then followed for 8 weeks after the 12-week treatment period. A blinded dermatologist, independent of the trial, then used standardized photographs to score the treated skin for wrinkles (on a 9-point scale measuring severity of wrinkles), uneven pigmentation and redness, plus an assessment of skin roughness was performed.

The results showed that both daily and biweekly treatments at all levels resulted in a significant improvement, of at least 1 point on the 9-point scale, for the group as a whole.

At treatment level 2, 4 weeks after the first treatment (week 16) 75% of subjects improved by 1 point on the 9-point scale for crow's feet, redness, nose-to-mouth lines, and uneven skin tone.

Infrared Light Technology

Deep heating by infrared light has been proven effective at tightening skin for up to 12 months after treatment. Collagen production is increased, which is said to occur for up to 3 or 4 months after treatment.

There are some very affordable infrared and red-light devices, with decent results for people on a limited budget. Some of them are coupled with vibration to increase blood circulation to the skin at the same time, particularly useful if you use it following a skin supplement.

Radio Frequency and Long Wavelengths

There are now multiple forms of radiofrequency therapies used in clinics to tighten loose skin around the face, neck and body. Thermage was introduced in 1999 in California. A study off 66 subjects showed an improvement in 84% of patients, when examined by an independent physician, six months after treatment.

IPL Laser

Intense pulsed light treatments have been used in clinics and at home for the treatment of body and face hair, to reduce thread veins and to reduce brown and red discolouration such as age marks, freckles, rosacea or pigmented scars.

It also stimulates the production of collagen and elastin, at the same wavelengths as used to treat brown and red discolouration (530-690 nm). Acne is treatment at shorter wavelengths of approximately 400 nm, whilst hair removal takes place at 750 nm. A lot of the devices on the market emit all of these, as the light contains a broad range of frequencies.

I have an IPL at home device that emits light across these wavelengths. I see it as my all-in-one leg-hair fighting, moustache zapping, freckle busting anti-wrinkle friend.

Section 4:

Natural Remedies, Nutrition, and Hydration

There's more to this than just skin, Jim

Exercise

Exercise is a great option to help us to tone up and to lose weight. A toned and lean appearance is the very essence of youth. As mentioned earlier, how much weight we tend to carry usually increases as we age, naturally this will form part of how others perceive our age. In addition, resistance training with weights, or even just our body weight, encourages our bones to increase in density, protecting us from the development of osteoporosis as we age.

Exercise can vary in intensity, depending on your preferences. Interval training is said to be an excellent, quick and intense way to shed some extra pounds of fat, whilst swimming is low impact and can achieve weight loss and toning as well. Yoga, Pilates and weight training can tighten your muscles, giving you a long, lean appearance. All are excellent options for maintaining a youthful and energised appearance.

I'm not going to provide a guide on these various types of exercise or routines, as there's an abundance of information out there already, you can't fail to miss it! Simply hit YouTube and search for videos at whatever level you prefer, or look for in-person classes at local sports centres.

Facial exercise

Facial exercises are an excellent way to build muscle volume, and keep the face taught. Not only this, but they boost circulation to the facial muscles and skin, delivering nutrients as they do so. They are also said to encourage collagen and elastic growth in the skin, although I am yet to see evidence for this.

Facial exercises work very much like regular exercise. In the same way that a weight-lifter or body-sculptor changes the shape of their muscles, so we can apply this to the muscles of the face. Less strenuous exercises with more repetitions can tone and tighten, whilst higher impact exercises can be used to create an increase in muscle volume. See below for an essential routine.

Essential facial exercise routine

Exercise 1 The Crow's Feet Buster:

Step 1: Create "V"s with your index and middle fingers

Step 2: Press the middle fingers into the inner corner of each eyebrow

Step 3: Lay the index fingers onto the face from the outer corner of each eyebrow down across the cheekbones

Step 4: Look up at the ceiling, raise your lower eyelids up and squint strongly for three seconds, then relax

Step 5: Repeat seven times

Exercise 2 Cheek Lifter

Step 1: Open your mouth and smile widely from your eyes and upper cheeks

Step 2: Hide your teeth with your lips. This is tricky but try your best!

Step 3: Keeping the hidden smile pose, tilt your head back, place your index finger on the chin, and open and close your jaw seven times. Keep your cheeks taught. You should feel the tightness in your upper cheeks

Step 4: Repeat three more times

Exercise 3 The Jowl Buster

Step 1: Tilt your head back gently so that you are looking at the ceiling, and push your lower jaw forward. You should feel a tightness across your neck

Step 2: Open and close your jaw, keeping your neck taught three times

Step 3: Stick out your lower jaw and hold, repetitively running your hand from your chin to the bottom of your neck. Hold for five seconds

Step 4: Repeat five times

Exercise 4 Marionette Line Beater

Step 1: Open your mouth wide and insert both index fingers into the insides of your cheeks

Step 2: Pull your fingers outwards so that you are stretching your cheeks apart

Step 3: Using the strength of your lips and your cheeks, pull your fingers back inwards, resisting the motion with your fingers as you do so

Step 4: Repeat three times and then hold for five seconds

Step 5: Repeat all steps seven times

Exercise 5 Peachy Cheeks

Step 1: Purse your lips and tighten the apples of your cheeks- a little like an over the top pout, or "duck face" selfie pose as some might see it.

Step 2: Using your index finger and middle finger, gently massage the apples of your cheeks in small circles. Apply enough pressure so that you can feel your cheek muscles working

Step 3: Continue for thirty seconds, stretch out the face and repeat three times

Boost Circulation

Boosting the circulation to our skin is a great way to deliver nutrients to the skin, and gives a youthful glow. This can be done with exercise, facial massage, or facial sauna.

If you combine a circulation boosting technique with your nutritional routine, consuming healthy nutrient-rich foods or supplements with water thirty minutes beforehand, you will be boosting your chances of delivering these nutrients directly to your skin.

A facial sauna can be as simple as boiling some water and pouring it into a bowl, placing a towel over your head and sitting with your face over the bowl. The steam heats your face, opening your pores and increasing the circulation to your skin. Your pores will cleanse themselves, and if you add the right ingredients, you can use a facial sauna to deep cleanse and purify the skin.

Purifying tea tree and menthol anti-bacterial steam

Step 1: Pour 2 litres of almost boiling water into a large bowl, in the position where you will be using it

Step 2: Add 5-6 drops each of tea tree oil and menthol

Step 3: Place your head over the bowl and cover your head and the bowl with a towel

Step 4: Sit for twenty minutes with your face in the steam. Be careful not to hold your face so close to the water that it feels as though it is being scorched by the steam, as this may damage the skin.

Doing this once a week for twenty minutes will not only help to boost circulation to the skin, but will also have the added benefit of deep cleansing the pores, encouraging them to open and release trapped sebum and oil.

After the steaming session, exfoliate using the blueberry, yoghurt and oatmeal scrub

Glowing complexions and youth

Colourful, glowing complexions are associated with health and youth, a handy tip to remember when applying makeup. This was demonstrated during a study that showed how increased yellow and red tones (combined this creates peachy/orangey tones) in two photographs of the same individual increased the perceived health and attractiveness of the same person considerably.

Applying a little blusher to the apples of the cheeks, the temples and at low levels around the face can work wonders if the blusher is a natural colour.

My natural skin tone is pale with blue undertones, and so I brighten my complexion with peachy cream blusher and golden-light highlighter at various points around my face, including the apples of my cheeks, around the eyes, under my bottom lip and on either side of my nose.
I keep this subtle, and never use a colour which is meant to be "dramatic," (such as bright pink) only natural, such as rose or peach.

Whatever your skin tone, finding a complimentary highlighter and blusher to give your face a flushed, plump and dewy look can work wonders for turning back the clock and how healthy you look in general.

Fish oils

I cannot get enough of how many benefits these incredible oils seem to show in an ever-increasing number of studies. There seems to be no end to the good news!

Studies have shown that these healthy oils, including omega 3, and 6 (but particularly omega 3), protect our heart health, boost our brain power, stabilize moods, prevent cancer, maintain our bone density and prevent macular degeneration.

They also slow down the inevitable DNA damage in cells. One study by the University of California found that the more omega 3 subjects ate, the slower this damage occurred. Subsequently, this is meant to deliver better protection from the aging process.

Drinking water

It has been touted for years that drinking more water will hydrate your skin, improving appearance and preventing aging. But is there any evidence behind it? This is debatable, mainly because the studies that say that it is true are single studies, which contradict other studies. The Mayoclinic, for example, cites that there is not enough evidence to say that drinking more water has any benefit to your skin.

On the other hand, if we look at the results of one study that says that there is a benefit, we see that the benefit is mostly to people that have lower daily water consumption. Adding 2 litres of water to the experimental group for one month, can increase the ability of the skin to snap back to its original shape after it is stretched.

Collagen Drinks

Collagen Gold was developed by Japanese scientists and is based on advanced understanding of the collagen used within our bodies, and particularly our skin.

A UK trial of 108 patients showed that after 6 weeks of drinking collagen gold there was a 27% decrease in deep wrinkles and after nine weeks the skin elasticity had increased by 20%.

It was found that taking the drink daily increased not only collagen and elastin but hyaluronic acid levels as well.

This drink is very expensive, and although I do take it, I tend to couple it together with when I am undergoing IPL and infrared light treatments on my face, and take it with omega 3 oils, so that it can have a maximum chance to have an effect.

Biotin (vitamin B7)

Biotin has been taken as a supplement for strong hair, nails and skin for many years. However, it is debated as to whether it is necessary to take in a supplement form. It has been shown to improve the keratin structure found in hair, skin and nails, but deficiency is rare.

Biotin has been proven to safely increase the growth of hair in women who have experienced temporary thinning. It is often found as part of hair, nail and skin supplements.

Imedeen

I was very surprised when I found Imedeen supplements. A supplement with proof-of-efficacy for anti-aging? Sounds like the stuff of quacks and con artists to me! And then I looked at the studies. I was rather impressed.

The supplements are expensive, but then, I'm quite vain and my skin has been noticeably softer since I started them about two months ago. However, I'm just as vulnerable to the placebo effect as the next person.

Several products are offered (of course) and I was very careful about reading up to see if there was a "cheaper" version for "younger" people which can sometimes be a trick to reduce the concentrations of the proven effective ingredients in (always trying to cut costs these businesses).

Imedeen Derma One is a product for those aged 30+ looking to "boost radiance," Imedeen Time Perfection is for those 40+ looking to "keep fine lines and wrinkles at bay" and Imedeen Prime Renewal is for those who are 50+ and trying to combat the effects of the menopause on their skin.

Honestly- at this point- this is all words. I'm also not going to be advised about which product to buy because of my age- because I'll take whichever one has been proven to be most effective for skin anti-aging- not the one the marketer wants me to buy which may well contain weaker, concentrations or completely different ingredients (I never said that it wasn't still a minefield when you're sorting through evidence trying to get a glimpse of the truth).

Skipping straight to the scientific documentation, Derma One has been the subject of 4 studies, ONE of which displays some carefully selected evidence to be displayed on the website- in this case cross-sections of skin. At month 0 a cross-section of skin showing collagen fibres.

At month 12 a cross-section of skin showing much thicker, denser skin and more collagen fibres. No other numerical information is available to show group comparisons. So, this image was of one subject who had the best improvement in skin density and collagen fibres.

Don't get me wrong- that's great! That's proof of efficacy for that one person- but it also suggests that this is the best result they had. It's not proof that it'll work anywhere nearly as well for you or me. And how does this cross-section of skin relate to real life wrinkles? The webpage doesn't mention wrinkles... at all…Next!

On the website, Imedeen Time Perfection seem to have had better results to display, because it looks as though they've decided to share study data that compares a treatment group with placebo. 6 scientific studies have been conducted, and the one they've selected to show on their website (and therefore must have the most impressive results) shows that at 12 weeks there is a 30% increase in moisture balance between Imedeen and placebo.

But hang on… there's no mention of how many people the graph data includes… so, it may just be the data pulled for one individual, who knows! Still, the product claims explicitly that this formulation has been shown to "increase dermal density, help improve skin quality and moisture balance and reduce the appearance of fine lines and wrinkles," which means, although we don't really know how much by as a group, we know that it does have some (even if very small) effect, or they would not be allowed to explicitly state it.

Imedeen Prime Renewal's page shows a graph of dermal density- again without showing the number of people in the graph sample size so we have no idea if this is the best performing individual, or the whole study group. The website states "The daily use of IMEDEEN Prime Renewal tablets has been shown to increase dermal density, help maintain skin firmness, help improve skin quality and moisture balance as well as reduce the appearance of fine lines and wrinkles"

I'm in a quandary. I seem to be the only person who's looking for robust evidence for anti-aging products (except for dermatologists who will have expensive subscriptions to dermatology journals, where they can pour over the trial design, and pick holes in the methodology).

And my end decision on this? I decided to give the Time Perfection formulation a go. I really plucked a choice from the air here, and taking a gamble on their appallingly thin (but very pretty) study data which is not filling me with confidence that I'll see any difference.

My reasoning- this choice has the most studies associated with it (a sign of higher investment?), and it specifically mentions reducing the appearance of fine lines and wrinkles, as well as increasing dermal density- whereas Derma One doesn't.

And if I don't notice any effect? Then I'll save my money and spend it on things where the evidence is clear.

Green Tea and Green Tea Extract

In 2003, it was reported by the International Journal of Vitamin and Nutritional Research that green tea extract delays collagen aging in mice. Whilst this is far from a human study meaning we have no evidence to suggest that this would be the same in humans, this would be an interesting development to look out for!

Green tea contains anti-oxidants, said to slow down the aging process as they absorb "free-radicals," highly reactive molecules that are created as part and parcel of our body's metabolism. These free radicals cause mutations which age not only our skin but the rest of our body tissues as well.

Anti-Oxidant Rich Foods

Anti-oxidants are not simply potential beneficial in skincare. Several studies have investigated the link between anti-oxidants found in bright, colourful foods such as blueberries, purple cabbage, blackberries, strawberries, carrots, and oranges and degenerative diseases such as Alzheimer's.

Many berries have high levels of antioxidants, with goji berries coming in at double the levels of blueberries. Dark chocolate also has high levels, as go pecans, artichokes kidney beans and cranberries. Antioxidants are often brightly coloured. You can enhance your diet not only by eating foods that are known to be high in anti-oxidants, but by ensuring that you eat a wide range of colours. Green spinach, orange carrots and red tomatoes all contain different anti-oxidants as well as different combinations of vitamins and minerals. A healthy diet should include a range of these nutrients.

Section 5:

Hair, Brows, Teeth, Lips, Neck and Muscle Tone

Maintaining Hair

As we age, our hair changes. Not only the hair on our heads, but also that of our eyebrows and eyelashes. Our hair colour is likely to fade in vibrancy before going grey, become less shiny due to a reduction in the production of serum from our scalp, and thin both in number and diameter of the hair shaft.

Head Hair

We can combat changes to our head hair can be in various ways. The dulling colour can be greatly improved using colour-rich hair dyes. I choose semi-permanent hair colour, to avoid damaging and drying my hair. These can also colour greys, although the grey hairs will emerge after several washes, so be warned!

In terms of increasing the shininess of our hair, there are some great products to choose from. I prefer serum, the sole purpose of which is to smooth down stray hairs and add a shiny surface layer to wet hair before you style it. It can also be used on dry hair once you have finished styling.

The golden rule with serum is that less is more, as this stuff can be super greasy. Hair spray and shine spray are also good options. Hair straighteners will straighten hairs into a smooth, uniform shape, making hair shinier, but always use heat protection spray to prevent permanent damage to the hair. Nothing will age your hair faster than broken, frizzy ends.

Biotin as part of a healthy skin, hair and nails supplement has also been shown to increase hair growth in women who have experienced temporary hair thinning, perhaps because of stress or dieting. See more in the supplements section.

Eyebrows

To me, eyebrows are one of the most important aspects of the face. The good news is that you can enhance them to have a real impact on how you look.

Eyebrows frame the face and are responsible for a great deal of our perceived attractiveness. I believe they act as indicators of both age and genetic health through colour, sparseness/fullness and shape.

Eyebrows should be well groomed. Specific tips on how to groom your eyebrows, and the perfect eyebrow shape will be included in my next book on signs of genetic health and fertility.

Studies have shown that thin, yet dark or "non-sparse" eyebrows are deemed the most attractive. As we age, the thickness and colour of our eyebrows diminish.   To   prevent   eyebrows appearing sparse I would recommend choosing an appropriate colour powder (be careful not to choose a colour that is too dark) and an eyebrow pencil, gel, pen or other product to define your brows. This will frame your face, give your face a boost of colour and fill in any gaps.

If you find you have gaps in your eyebrows from over-plucking the hairs can be encouraged by application of an eyebrow serum, such as "Rapid Brow." This serum has been clinically proven to increase eyebrow density up to 108% in 60 days. A similar product can be bought for eyelashes, which causes lashes to grow up to 50% longer in 60 days.

Dying your eyebrows using specialist dyes can also be effective. I'll let you into a little secret, the best product I've found to this job is actually Just for Men moustache dye! It works in less than five minutes and afterwards I have the brows of a young Brooke Shields (alright, maybe I'm exaggerating). Bragging aside, the first time I tried it I looked more like Tom Selleck. You have been warned, try it, but the first time you apply it, remember that less is more!

Semi-permanent eyebrow tattooing, microblading, pencilling, powder, or eyebrow gel, are all options to play with depending on your budget and how much time you want to spend in the mornings. If you've never had your eyebrows professionally shaped, trying this will show you what a huge difference they can make to your overall youthful look.

Receding gums and yellowing teeth

Naturally as we age, our teeth discolour and our gums often recede. These signs of age can be reduced with good oral hygiene, and/or professional help. A good hygienist will help combat gum recession by cleaning under the gum-line and allowing the gums to heal. Brushing your teeth twice a day is essential, and using dental floss is a good way to maintain gum health.

In terms of preventing discolouration, teeth can be whitened professionally by a cosmetic dentist, or at home using DIY teeth whitening kits. If you choose to whiten your teeth at home, always make sure you follow the instructions and don't keep any treatments on longer than the recommended time. Sensitivity of the teeth following whitening can be excruciatingly painful so always be careful! I once left a DIY whitening strip on longer than the recommended time and experienced flashes of pain throughout the following day.

To maintain teeth at their best, or to remove stains, baking soda is a cheap and effective home remedy. Simply apply to the teeth using a toothbrush and leave for 2 minutes.

Red wine, coffee and tea are all drinks that will discolour and age your teeth. If you can't resist them, at least resist them during the week following any tooth whitening that you undertake- as it will be then that your teeth are at their most porous, and will uptake stains far more easily than usual. There are products which seal the teeth and prevent them from taking up stains, that help to prolong the whitening effect.

Facial and Neck Muscle Stimulation

Loss of muscle tone in the face as we age can create sags, bags, jowls and droopiness. Electro muscle stimulation (EMS) technology is well-known for toning areas of the body such as the stomach and arms. An electrical current stimulated the muscles to contract, resulting in exercise whilst passively wearing an EMS device such as a belt.

There are also such devices for the face, and these are available in the form of a "headset," such as the Slendertone, electrodes that allow you to target specific muscles, such as the Cleo Q, or a pair of electrodes to hold against the face or neck such as the Rio 60 second Facial toner.

Let's look at Slendertone Face. A 12-week clinical trial showed an average increase of 18.6% *muscle volume*, with a maximum increase of 46%. There were no results for whether *fat content* was lowered, however, and as fatty pads in the face are a key factor in "youthfulness" this is a key as to whether the device would increase of decrease perceived age.

Personally, I wouldn't use it as described until I feel that I have already lost considerable muscle tone or cheek volume, as I would not want to "exercise my fat pads away" (which is what makes you look young). According to one study by a Harley Street cosmetic surgeon described in the next section, this should not happen until age 40 to 50. The changed in volume then occur swiftly, over the course of roughly 1 year.

EMS can also be used to tighten the chin, and there are also devices which can be used for this purpose. The Rio 60 Second Neck Toner showed an average 33% increase in tone and firmness in the neck after 15 days involving 73 women.

Section 6:

Avoiding aging

Be aware of what accelerates aging,
before you start trying to stop it!

Age Spurts: Dieting and Stress

Age spurts- they're real! Don't get caught unprepared. One informative study Mr Grover, a cosmetic surgeon in London has found some fascinating insights into aging spurts and triggers.

Mr Grover found that some parts of our life stories can cause rapid accelerations, or spurts, in aging to the face. The biggest culprits are yo-yo dieting, significant weight loss, bereavement, divorce and stress.

He followed 118 women aged 40 to 45 for up to 9 years (on average 7.2 years), and took annual measurements of various parts of the face. He then looked to see the speed at which the face aged over the years, and took lifestyle factors and life events into account, to see whether events in life affect facial aging.

The face was assessed in thirds, and brow height, fat volume in the cheeks, and the depth of the nasolabial fold and jowl thickness were all measured.

It was found that ageing is gradual in the brow, forehead, jowls and jawline, but that in the mid-third of the face aging is far more dramatic. Up to 35% of cheek volume can be lost within one year.

The most significant factor driving age spurts was yo-yo dieting, with the loss of more than 11lbs during one year. Mr Grover accounted this to the stretching and relaxing of ligaments which support facial soft tissue. Other triggers include stress and trauma, such as that experienced from a redundancy, divorce, illness or bereavement.

Stress is thought to speed up the aging process in a number of ways. The stress hormone, cortisol, causes a rise in blood sugar, blood pressure and reduces immune system resistance to infection. One study also shows that cortisol suppresses the activation of an important enzyme, telomerase, responsible for preserving the "youth" of all of our body cells.

Telomerase prevents the shortening of tiny "clocks" at the end of our chromosomes called telomeres, which prevent loss or damage to our genetic material during cell reproduction. Every time a cell divides part of the telomere cap is lost, and it becomes shorter. Whilst cells with long telomeres live longer, short telomeres have been linked with a wide range of diseases such as coronary heart disease and osteoporosis. Those of us who are exposed to chronic stress have been found to have shorter telomeres than those who are not. For example, one study found that mothers of severely and chronically sick children had shorter telomeres when compared with other women.

We can consider our lifestyles an important factor in holding back- or accelerating- the clock. If you're trying to lose weight, lose it gradually. You may have to compromise between your weight-loss goals and your anti-aging goals to a degree, as too much weight loss could leave you feeling unhappy with the effects on your facial tautness, so it is best to monitor changes to your face carefully when on a diet.

In terms of stress- although many of the most stressful life events are not under our control, we can at least prepare and fight against them by taking steps to limit our stress wherever possible.

Although beauty may be the furthest thing from our minds when we are stressed, we may also wish to combat the detrimental effects on our looks with a good skincare, lifestyle and nutrient regime to protect our health as well as our skin.

So, what are the other environmental causes of skin-aging?

Ultra Violet Light

The most well-known aging influence on our skin is ultra violet light, or sunlight is responsible for up to 80% of skin aging. Most of the wrinkles and discolouration that we consider a normal part of aging are caused by UV light. Fibres within the skin, known as elastin are broken down at an accelerated rate, and the skin begins to wrinkle and sag.

According to the World Health Organization-there is "no such thing as a healthy tan!" because the melanin produced in the skin as a reaction to UV light is a sign that your skin has been damaged. So, what is going on beneath the surface? Several factors are at play here- UVB stimulates the reproduction of cells in the outer layer of the skin, thickening it.

UVA penetrates more deeply and damages the connective tissue within the skin, so that it loses its elasticity, resulting in wrinkles and sagginess. Often there is a localised over-production of melanin, as seen in freckles or "sun-spots" which often appear as we age as a sign of damage sustained in earlier years. The skin dries out giving it a course and leathery appearance.

To protect our skin from damage there are several simple precautions we can take. Limit the amount of sun exposure you receive, particularly between the hours of 10am and 4pm when the sun is at its strongest. It is also useful to look up the local UV index in your area on days when you expect to be outside, which will alert you to particularly high levels of UV to watch out for.

Hats, and sunglasses that provide 99 to 100 percent UVA and UVB protection will keep your face eyes safe from damage. Loose-fitting clothes that cover the shoulders and chest will also prevent these areas showing signs of sun damage.

Finally, applying a broad-spectrum SPF 15+ sunscreen regularly whilst outside will greatly help to reduce sun damage. In case you need to be told- don't use sunbeds or tanning parlours! You might enjoy your tan in the short-term but in the long-term your skin will not thank you.

Sugar

Sugar speeds up the destruction of collagen and elastin in the skin, accelerating the aging process through a process called glycation. It binds to the proteins so that they become brittle and break. But it doesn't stop there, glycation also causes mutations resulting in inflammation and even more damage to the collagen and elastin.
Whilst anti—oxidants such as those in green tea, blueberries or purple cabbage may help reduce glycation, the most effective way to stop it is to remove processed sugar from your diet, and switch over to eating complex carbohydrates.

Smoking

Most of us have heard that smoking is bad for the skin. But few people know more than that. Not only is smoking associated with premature facial wrinkling, but it is also associated with poor wound healing.

The results of one 2002 study by Knuutinen *et al.* showed how smoking affects collagen synthesis, and the rate at which the "extracellular matrix" renews itself (which is a collection of molecules that are secreted by cells to provide support and structure to the surrounding cells).

The study found that smoking decreases the rate of "type I" and "type III" collagen production in the skin. It was also found that certain molecules within the extracellular matrix varied between smokers and non-smokers, and that the regeneration rate of the matrix was also lower in smokers.

A particularly interesting study in 2013 looked at the difference in facial aging between identical twins with different smoking histories. Bags beneath the eyes, wrinkles on the upper lids and jowls were all found to be noticeably worse amongst the twins with greater than 5 years difference in smoking duration. An incentive if ever you needed one to pack in the cigarettes once and for all!

Alcohol

Alcohol is generally dehydrating, and dehydrates the skin. If you're partial to a few cheeky drinks on a Friday evening (as I am) you might have noticed your skin is particularly dry the next day. You don't need to cut out alcohol entirely, but it is best to keep alcohol intake within moderation, intersperse alcoholic drinks with soft drinks, and drink plenty of water to keep your body and skin hydrated.

It's also worth mentioning that heavy drinking over time can also lead to reddening of the cheeks, burst blood vessels and rosacea- not a good look for the fashion-conscious.

Section 7:

Building Your Youthful Routine

How old would you feel if you didn't know how old you were?

Putting Theory into Practice

There are many techniques that you can use to help hold back the tide of time. Nothing will last forever, of course, but we can give it a damn good try! You can combat aging from the inside, from the outside, in your sleep, as part of your daily routine, with your clothing choices- just about any time and any place.

A basic moisturiser will do a good job of hydrating the skin and preventing and even slightly reducing skin wrinkling. There are several topical skin creams that have been proven to maintain or improve skin quality, and the most effective is not the most expensive.

Using a facial muscle stimulator can really prevent muscle loss or wastage between the ages of 40 and 50, but because the facial fat pads are key to making us look young, they should really be used with caution.

Light and various types of radiation have demonstrated proven results that will turn back the hands of time by stimulating or damaging the skin. Fraxel, IPL and infrared options can all be used at home, with very cheap, proven infrared options out there for people on limited budgets.

If I need to lose weight, am going through stress or hardship, I will keep myself topped up from the inside with the vitamins and minerals that my skin and body needs in the form of Imedeen supplements, plenty of omega 3 oils and fresh fruit and vegetables.

Easiest of all has got to be sleeping on a Cupron copper-infused pillowcase to reduce eye wrinkles by 10%. You really can't get easier than sleeping your "wisdom" away!

On the next pages, I have included an organiser to help you amalgamate the tips from this book into a workable routine. I have summarized all the sections and tips in this book. with a place for notes, budget, and when you would fit each into your routine.

Lastly, I have included a "schedule" table for you to pull together a convenient "to do" list for your new routine, to help you turn it into a reality. Research suggests that it takes approximately three to four weeks to create a new habit, and so if you can keep up the routine for this long, you are well on your way to success!

Putting tips to good use…

Section 1: Understanding Research

Tip	When/how can I use this?
If there is real proof behind a product it will use the words "clinically proven to work" or "proven to work,"	
Do your homework on a product before you buy, look for a randomized controlled clinical trial- which should be "double blinded" and tell you exactly what the benefits of the product are	
Approval ratings or consumer opinions are NOT evidence of	

efficacy

The biases in consumer opinion polls include:
Positivity bias (people are mostly very eager to please)
The placebo effect (people see or believe in change)
There is often no basis for objective comparison

Wrinkling skin, grey hair, lip height, facial sun-damage, and recession of the hairline all increase perception of age

Hair thinning was found to be caused by environmental causes such as stress, dieting, illness or pregnancy, and tends to reverse when the cause is removed

Section 2: Skincare Products and Moisturizers

Tip	When/how can I use this?
Basic moisturizers work quite well, because they boost hydration levels	
Few topical creams that boost collagen and elastin have high enough levels of active ingredients to actually work	
AHA moisturizers should contain at least eight percent lactic, tartaric or glycolic acid to treat prematurely aged skin, and be applied twice daily	

Metrixyl moisturizers sold by Boots have solid evidence that they reduce wrinkles and repair sun damage to a greater degree than basic moisturizers

Tretinoin (vitamin A) and Retinol are the only FDA approved topical treatments for wrinkles, and require a prescription rather than being available over the counter.

Ambiguous claims, or relying solely on opinion-poll data, mean there is likely to be no scientific evidence that a product works any better than a basic moisturizer

Section 3: Tools and Devices

Tip	When/how can I use this?
Copper infused fabrics increase collagen growth in the skin. After eight weeks using a Cupron pillowcase skin wrinkles were reduced by 10%	
Fraxel at-home technology either reduced fine lines, evened skin tone or improved texture in most women tested	
Infrared light treatments increase collagen for up to twelve months after treatment	
Radio frequency technology is available in clinics and tightened the skin of most participants tested	

IPL laser can be used at home and can reduce pigmentation, rosacea, hair growth, and stimulate collagen production

Section 4: Natural Remedies

Tip	When/how can I use this?
Exercise can help us appear younger by toning us up	
Reducing our BMI to be in line with younger people can have the effect of reducing perceived age, but as dieting is also likely to reduce facial volume, small weight-loss goals may be more effective than large ones	
Boosting circulation gives a colourful glow to the skin and delivers nutrients	
Using blusher and highlighter on our cheeks can make us appear healthy, vibrant and youthful	

Facial exercises can tighten the facial muscles, lifting sagging tissue improving the appearance of the face
Omega 3 oils have been preliminarily linked with slower DNA damage in cells, potentially protecting us from the aging process
Drinking more water can help boost skin hydration levels in those that are not sufficiently hydrated
Collagen drinks have solid evidence to show that they can decrease wrinkles and improve skin elasticity
Biotin, a common component of hair and skin supplements has inconclusive evidence as to whether it improves the quality

of our skin, hair or nails in most people
Imedeen supplements have evidence that they work in some people, but it is impossible to objectively assess the extent of this and average effects on those who take it
Foods rich in anti-oxidants such as green tea, blueberries and purple cabbage may slow down the aging process

Section 5: Hair, Brows, Teeth, Lips, Neck and Muscle Tone

Tip	When/how can I use this?
Hair colour dulls as	

we age, so increasing the vibrancy of hair using colour-rich hair dyes can help reduce perceived age

Eyebrows become less dense and vibrant as we age. There are products that increase the density of eyebrows effectively. Also, defining, thickening or darkening them can reduce perceived age

Eyelash length can be increased using effective products that stimulate their growth

Yellowing teeth and receding gums are a sign of age. Good oral health, avoiding staining and whitening our teeth can remove years and give us a healthy appearance

Facial and neck muscle stimulation can effectively tighten sagging neck skin and build muscle volume in the face. Beware of overuse in the face, as it may reduce the youthful fatty pads, which will decrease volume, leading to sagging

Section 6: Avoiding Aging

Tip	When/how can I use this?
Continuous dieting is the biggest cause of accelerated facial aging	
UV light is responsible for up to 80% of skin aging, making sun protection a vital part of a skincare regime, particularly in summer.	
To reduce sun damage, avoid sun exposure between the hours of 10 am to 4pm when the sun is at its strongest	
Choose a broad-brimmed hat to protect your face from UV light in the sun	
Choose sunglasses with 99-100% UVA	

and UVB protection to shield your eyes from damage

Select a sun cream that reduces both UVA and UVB effectively with at least SPF 15+

Sugar speeds up the production of collagen and elastic, accelerating the aging process

Smoking accelerates skin aging and reduces wound healing by reducing the production of collagen

Alcohol is dehydrating, so rehydrate throughout the night and next day if you're going to partake!

Bibliography

Section 1: Marketing Fluff vs. Proof

1. The skin care market: https://goo.gl/o4gyzO
2. Clinical trials and medical research: http://www.nhs.uk/Conditions/Clinical-trials/Pages/Definition.aspx
3. 9 Skincare Myths: https://goo.gl/NVksWy
4. Why some Women Look Young for their Age: https://goo.gl/49OhdZ

Section 2: Skincare Products and Moisturizers

2.1 The effects of basic moisturizer

1. Review of Skin Aging and Dry Skin: Journal of Dermatology: https://goo.gl/m2cGgf
2. The influences of skin visco-elasticity, hydration level and aging on the formation of wrinkles: https://goo.gl/tc0RUA
3. Mayoclinic: Moisturizers Options for Skin: https://goo.gl/Z5tiVf

2.2 Alpha-Hydroxy Acid Moisturizer

1. Alpha-Hydroxy Acids: WebMD: https://goo.gl/k5Njpr

2. Effects of alpha-hydroxy acids on the human skin: Journal of Dermatology: https://goo.gl/3kAjQF
3. NeoStrata Face Cream Plus (15% Glycolic Acid): https://goo.gl/UCJV0k
4. Peter Thomas Roth Glycolic Acid 10% Moisturizer: https://goo.gl/oZksi0
5. Peaches & Crème AHA 4% Moisturizer: https://goo.gl/l0Cvvv

2.3 Metrixyl Moisturizers

1. Metrixyl 3000 Study: https://goo.gl/QzjBbx
2. Protect and Perfect Advanced Serums: https://goo.gl/QPb0gc
3. BBC News: Proof face creams beat wrinkles: https://goo.gl/xu9lFT

2.4 Tretinoin and Retinol

1. Retinoid creams: WebMD: https://goo.gl/Aw6bXH
2. Tretinoin Cream: Drugs.com: https://goo.gl/7xFegn
3. Imedeen Supplements: https://goo.gl/91jEjh

Section 3: Tools and Devices

3.1 Cupron Pillowcase

1. Cupron: 10% Wrinkle Reduction: https://goo.gl/RvJGj3
2. The Cupron Difference: https://goo.gl/lLqnzj

3.2 Anti-Aging Laser Technology

1. Fraxel: Philips ReAura: https://goo.gl/Tgndlx
2. Fraxel: Tria Age-Defying Laser: https://goo.gl/jyJzN1
3. Infrared and Radiofrequency: Technology report for the American Society for Dermatological Surgery: https://goo.gl/93NCm3
4. Intense Pulsed Light: https://goo.gl/EHcxyL

Section 4: Natural Remedies, Nutrition and Hydration

1. Hydrated Skin: Does drinking water help? https://goo.gl/tjg1OD
2. Drinking water: affects human skin hydration and biomechanics: https://goo.gl/XGAOOT
3. Omega 3: https://goo.gl/fA502S
4. Biotin: https://goo.gl/kqwsVJ
5. Imedeen Supplements: https://goo.gl/JKSVwI
6. Collagen Gold: https://goo.gl/TwByN0
7. Green Tea Extract: https://goo.gl/ug5jUK

Section 5: Hair, Brows, Teeth, Lips, Neck and Muscle Tone

5.1 Eyelashes and Eyebrows

Rapid Lash: https://goo.gl/B3ACwi
Rapidbrow: https://goo.gl/Q1Lg8b

5.2 Facial Muscle Stimulation

Slendertone Face for Women: https://goo.gl/XqLTL7
Rio Beauty Facial Toners: https://goo.gl/9W3Shd

Section 6: Avoiding Aging

1. How your face reveals the traumas you've been through by ageing faster: goo.gl/zBF6EW
2. Sugar: https://goo.gl/iTA1TN
3. Sun-exposure and skin cancer: https://goo.gl/3c8UUK
4. Sun protection: https://goo.gl/oKZgjC
5. Smoking affects collagen synthesis and extracellular matrix turnover in human skin: https://goo.gl/rIS5rL
6. How alcohol affects your appearance: https://goo.gl/6Y5fkZ

About the Author

In 2016 Rachel Knight decided to use her master's degree in clinical research, and her experience of writing medical and scientific materials, for something good. She quit her corporate job in medical communications (producing materials that solely benefited pharmaceutical companies) and started writing to help people.

By sticking with her personal brand of evidence-based, scientific research, translated into "human" language, her whole world changed. She became location independent and discovered a new, immensely rewarding world of giving other people information that could potentially really make a difference in their lives.

As well as her master's degree in clinical research she has a bachelor's degree in physics with astrophysics. Half of her childhood was spent in the Bahamas before she returned to England, studied and traveled the world.

After several years spent working in South Korea, Spain, and the Netherlands, she went to London where she worked for five years serving pharmaceutical companies in healthcare communications agencies.

Having become location independent, she now spends much of her time in Italy and finally loves life again- something she whole-heartedly believes everyone deserves to do.

Books by Rachel Knight

Little-Known Secrets of ADHD. The Surprising Upside You Haven't Been Told **(excerpt to follow)**

Anti-Aging Skincare Secrets: The Beauty Scientist's Guide to Skincare

Bladder Cancer for Patients and Families: Guidance, Patient Experiences and Practical Resources

Colon Cancer 101 for Patients: Empowered in our Fight against Bowel Cancer

Diabetes and Foot Care for Patients: Essential tips to salvage your feet

46 Skincare Secrets to Get Rid of Wrinkles

Excerpt from:

Little-Known Secrets of ADHD

I decided to write this book when an interesting thought struck me:

Every successful entrepreneurial person I know has ADHD or ADHD tendencies.

Upon further investigation, I found out that ADHD isn't just prevalent amongst relatively normal, interesting people, it's also prevalent amongst the pinnacles of human achievement. Gold-medal-winning Olympic swimmer Michael Phelps channelled his energy into training, racking up 14 golds at the Athens and Beijing Olympics. He and his mother partially attribute his success to ADHD.

Albert Einstein is thought to have had ADHD, which is one reason why his genius wasn't recognised within the education system. Colossally successful entrepreneurs Sir Richard Branson (Founder of Virgin and Adventurer), Ingvar Kamprad (Founder of Ikea) and David Neeleman (Founder of JetBlue) all attribute their achievements to be partially *because* of their ADHD, rather than despite it.[1]

But it doesn't stop at entrepreneurialism and genius, it also applies to creative people. Emma Watson was diagnosed as a child and after finding fame on screen has found passion to tirelessly advocate women's rights around the globe. Grammy-winning musician Justin Timberlake reports himself to have ADD and OCD. This may be one reason he has the energy and drive to not only be a singer-songwriter but a restaurateur, tequila distiller, NBA part-owner, record executive and clothier.[2-4]

Digging a little deeper, I was no longer surprised to find that people with ADHD are 300% more likely to start their own businesses. When an ADHD'er finds their sweet-spot, it seems like magic can happen. In fact, it appears that often someone with ADHD can do *anything that deeply captures their interest.*

How could this be? Wasn't ADHD meant to be a bad thing? How could it be that many of the most successful people in history, and the most vivacious people I personally know (demonstrating success on both the macro and micro-level) seem to be thriving when they display the attributes of a disorder? In comparison to many of my non-ADHD friends- I don't mean to be rude- but the ADHD'ers tend to shine as beacons of inspiration.

Everywhere they go they're greeted with wonder at how they manage to achieve so much, or how they're living such exciting lives. At the risk of offending the rest of my friends and colleagues, they're the most engaging bunch I could imagine. There would be no hesitation if my fairy godmother asked me what kind of life I would prefer to lead, if I could pick between the two groups (ADHD'ers or non-ADHD'ers).

Because my previous career was spent serving pharmaceutical companies, I want to know specifically if the medical community has done ADHD a disservice.

I spent five years working in drug advertising, medical education, clinical trial recruitment and patient observation. I understand very well how disease awareness campaigns are created- with one objective from the main sponsor- to sell more drugs.

Pharma work hand-in-hand with charities and educational institutions to give their materials credibility. But let us make no mistake, negative aspects of diseases sell drugs, whilst positive aspects sell nothing.

So, my question again: has the medical community done those with ADHD a disservice?

To satisfy my curiosity about what was going on, I decided to interview successful people with ADHD, and publish their thoughts in this book, to see what lessons could be learnt. In particular, I wanted to answer the following questions:

What benefits and challenges have they met and overcome? How has ADHD affected them? How did they find success? Why did they lead such unusual lives? What made them start their own businesses or work for themselves?

As medical doctor and entrepreneur, Mo- who has moderate inattentive ADHD- explained, a normal person "who has no technical or specific knowledge of ADHD, who has been hearing about it in the media, is going to look at it as a disease. Which in many situations it is, but they won't see the positive aspects of it, because that's not the side that's advertised."

Can the positive side be harnessed?

One thing became abundantly clear during the interviews. These people have passion for what they do oozing from their pores. Perhaps not everyone, in everything that they do, but when it comes to their areas of interest, they had me drawn in, hooked, and carried away with their enthusiasm.

I can't help but wonder if these are typical ADHD'ers, or some kind of atypical, super-human subgroup. The truth is, that question can never be answered. As anecdotal evidence, there can be no statistical conclusions drawn about whether this sample is representative of a wider population. But even if it's not representative of the ADHD community as-a-whole, I love the way that there are many people who are a living testament that the accepted "norm" is often wrong. The idea that ADHD is some kind of terrible affliction, or a sentence that will ruin your life, in their cases, is simply not true. For them, despite the numerous challenges and difficulties being faced- particularly during their school years and early careers- the outcome has been quite the opposite. The strengths of ADHD have left them at a positive advantage over much of the population, in terms of pursuing their own goals and living life unashamedly on their own terms.

Their chosen lifestyles work *with* the ADHD brain, harnessing its vigilance for interesting, dopamine-inducing activities. They have allowed their addictive tendencies to fall on pursuits that were productive and made them happy.

This book is a protest, *against* the abundant literature published by pharma that discusses almost all aspects of ADHD as "problems." It focuses instead on how to look at the flip side of the coin and celebrates how people with ADHD creatively forge their own paths.

This positive approach is favoured over the task of how to make an ADHD'er fit into the glove of a "normal" life. Or how to help them do their homework, not answer back or pay their bills on time (there is enough material written on surmounting these challenges). In fact, we learn how some of our interviewees have avoided a situation where they were forced into a shoe that didn't fit, and in breaking free re-discovered their unique identity.

That said, this is not a thesis, research study or statistical summary of evidence on ADHD. It doesn't intend to tell you what to think, or get involved in the politics of whether to medicate, whether to call ADHD a superpower, learning disability or a disorder. It's simply some anecdotal inspiration to highlight how there are two sides to this story. In the words of doctor Mo (and I'll be calling him that for the entirety of this book, don't you know):

> "When you're researching always stick to the facts. It's good to learn about things from different sources, [such as this book, for example] but it's very important to look at what the recent research says. It's good to keep an evidence-based approach."

Caveats aside, our ADHD superstars are unafraid, unabashed, and possess the tenacity to get things done. You'll see that the energy that is common amongst ADHD'ers, is so often admired by others.

Leave a review…

If you enjoyed this book, found it useful or otherwise then I'd really appreciate it if you would post a short review. I do read all the reviews personally so that I can continually write what people are wanting.

Thanks for your support!

Get in touch…

If you would like to receive news of giveaways and new releases, please email me at rachel.knight.books@gmail.com and I'll add you to my readers list.